Beginners Plant Based Cookbook

100 Life-Changing Plant-Based Recipes

Nina R. Dalrymple

Contents

Chapter 1

Introduction

Morning Kasha with Mushrooms

(Ready in about 30 minutes | Servings 2)

Per serving : Calories: 446; Fat: 29g; Carbs: 1g; Protein: 6g

Ingredients

1 cup water

1/2 cup buckwheat groats, toasted

Sea salt and ground black pepper, to taste

2 tablespoons olive oil

1 cup button mushrooms, sliced\s2 tablespoons scallions, chopped\s1 garlic clove, minced

1 small avocado, pitted, peeled and sliced\s1 tablespoon fresh lemon juice

Directions

In a saucepan, bring the water and buckwheat to a boil. Immediately turn the heat to a

simmer and continue to cook for about 20 minutes. Season with sea salt and ground black pepper to taste.

Then, heat the olive oil in a nonstick skillet, over medium-high heat. Sauté the mushrooms, scallions and garlic for about 4 minutes or until they've softened.

Spoon the kasha into two serving bowls; top each serving with the sautéed mushroom mixture.

Garnish with avocado, add a few drizzles of fresh lemon juice and serve immediately. Bon appétit!

Tomato Tofu Scramble\s(Ready in about 15 minutes | Servings 3) Per serving : Calories: 399; Fat: 4g; Carbs: 3g; Protein: 3g

Ingredients

2 tablespoons olive oil

2 garlic cloves, minced\s12 ounces extra-firm tofu

1 medium-sized tomato, diced

2 tablespoons nutritional yeast

Kosher salt and ground black pepper, to taste

1/2 teaspoon red pepper flakes, crushed

A pinch of seaweed flakes

3 tablespoons soy milk, unsweetened

1 medium-sized avocado, pitted, peeled and sliced

Directions

Heat the olive oil in a nonstick skillet over a moderate flame. Then, sauté the garlic, tofu and tomato, crumbling the tofu with a fork, for about 8 minutes

Add in the nutritional yeast, salt, black pepper, red pepper, seaweed flakes and soy milk. Continue to sauté an additional 2 minutes.

Divide the scramble between three serving plates, garnish with avocado and serve. Bon appétit!

Spring Onion Flat Bread (Ready in about 30 minutes | Servings 3)

Per serving : Calories: 219; Fat: 5g; Carbs: 2g; Protein: 3g

Ingredients 1 cup all-purpose flour 1/2 teaspoon baking powder

1/4 teaspoon sea salt 1/2 cup warm water

1 cup spring onions, chopped

Sea salt and ground black pepper, to taste

1/2 teaspoon garlic powder

1/2 teaspoon cayenne pepper

1/2 teaspoon dried thyme

3 teaspoons olive oil

Directions

Thoroughly combine the flour, baking powder and salt in a mixing bowl. Gradually add in

the water until the dough comes together.

Add in the spring onions and spices and knead the dough one more time.

Divide the dough into three balls; flatten each ball to create circles.

Heat 1 teaspoon of the olive oil in a frying pan over a moderately high flame. Fry the first bread, turning it over to promote even cooking; fry it for about 9 minutes or until golden brown.

Repeat with the remaining oil and dough. Bon appétit!

Chocolate Granola Bars (Ready in about 40 minutes | Servings 12) Per serving : Calories: 229; Fat: 4g; Carbs: 9g; Protein: 1g

Ingredients 1 1/3 cups old-fashioned oats

1/2 cup fresh dates, pitted and mashed

1/2 cup dried cherries

1/3 cup agave syrup

1/3 cup almond butter, room temperature

2 tablespoons coconut oil, melted

1/2 cup almonds

1/2 cup walnuts

1/4 cup pecans

1/2 teaspoon allspice

A pinch of salt

A pinch of grated nutmeg

1/2 cup dark chocolate chunks

Directions

In a mixing bowl, thoroughly combine the oats, dates and dried cherries.

Add in the agave syrup, almond butter and coconut oil. Stir in the nuts, spices and chocolate.

Press the mixture into a lightly greased baking dish. Transfer it to your refrigerator for about

30 minutes.

Slice into 12 even bars and store in airtight containers. Enjoy!

Mexican-Style Omelet (Ready in about 15 minutes | Servings 2)

Per serving : Calories: 329; Fat: 4g; Carbs: 2g; Protein: 9g

Ingredients 2 tablespoons olive oil

1 small onion, chopped

2 Spanish peppers, deseeded and chopped

1/2 cup chickpea flour

1/2 cup water

3 tablespoons rice milk, unsweetened

2 tablespoons nutritional yeast

Kala namak salt and ground black pepper, to taste

1/2 teaspoon dried Mexican oregano

1/4 cup salsa

Directions

Heat the olive oil in a frying pan over medium-high flame. Once hot, sauté the onion and

peppers for about 3 minutes until tender and aromatic.

Meanwhile, whisk the chickpea flour with the water, milk, nutritional yeast, salt, black pepper and dried Mexican oregano.

Then, pour the mixture into the frying pan.

Cook for about 4 minutes. Turn it over and cook for an additional 3 to 4 minutes until set. Serve with salsa and enjoy!

Breakfast Cranberry and Coconut Crisp

(Ready in about 30 minutes | Servings 10)

Per serving : Calories: 209; Fat: 5g; Carbs: 2g; Protein: 5g

Ingredients 1/2 cup rye flakes

1/2 cup rolled oats 1/2 cup spelt flakes

1/2 cup walnut halves

1 cup flaked coconut

1/3 teaspoon salt

1/2 teaspoon ground cloves

1/2 teaspoon ground cardamom

1 teaspoon cinnamon

1 teaspoon vanilla extract

1/3 cup coconut oil, at room temperature

1/2 cup maple syrup

3 cups cranberries

Directions

Begin by preheating your oven to 340 degrees. Spritz a baking pan with a nonstick oil.

Arrange the cranberries in the bottom of your pan.

Mix the remaining Ingredients until everything is well incorporated. Spread the mixture over the cranberries.

Bake in the preheated oven for about 35 minutes or until the top is golden brown. 4. Serve at room temperature. Bon appétit!

Authentic French Toast with Strawberries (Ready in about 20 minutes | Servings 5)

Per serving : Calories: 296; Fat: 9g; Carbs: 3g; Protein: 9g

Ingredients 1 cup coconut milk

1/4 teaspoon sea salt 1/2 teaspoon ground cinnamon

1 teaspoon vanilla extract

1/2 teaspoon ground cardamom

1 French baguette, sliced

2 tablespoons peanut oil

2 ounces fresh strawberries, hulled and sliced

4 tablespoons confectioners' sugar

Directions

In a mixing bowl, thoroughly combine the milk, salt, cinnamon, vanilla and cardamom.

Dip each slice of bread into the milk mixture until well coated on all sides.

Preheat the peanut oil in a frying pan over medium-high heat. Cook for about 3 minutes on each side, until golden brown.

Serve the French toast with the strawberries and confectioners' sugar. Bon appétit!

Simple Wafers for Breakfast

(Serves 8) | Ready in 30 minutes

Serves: 1 288 calories, 1 gram of fat, 3 gram of carbohydrates, and 4 gram of protein

14 cup rice flour (ingredients)

1/2 cup potato starch + 1/4 cup tapioca flour

1 cup oats (instant)

1 teaspoon baking powder

1/2 teaspoon baking soda

1 pinch sea salt

1/2 teaspoon vanilla essence

1/2 teaspoon cinnamon

1 ½ cups oat milk

1 teaspoon apple cider vinegar

1/3 cup coconut oil, softened

1/3 cup maple syrup

Directions

Preheat a waffle iron according to the manufacturer's instructions.

In a mixing bowl, thoroughly combine the flour, potato starch, instant oats, baking powder,

baking soda, salt, vanilla and cinnamon.

Gradually add in the milk, whisking continuously to avoid lumps. Add in the apple cider vinegar, coconut oil and maple syrup. Whisk again to combine well.

Beat until everything is well blended.

Ladle 1/2 cup of the batter into the preheated iron and cook according to manufacturer instructions, until your wafers are golden. Repeat with the remaining batter. 6. Serve with toppings of choice. Bon appétit!

Traditional Ukrainian Blinis\s(Ready in about 1 hour | Servings 6) Per serving : Calories: 138; Fat: 7g; Carbs: 9g; Protein: 4g

Ingredients\s1 teaspoon yeast\s1 teaspoon brown sugar

3/4 cup oat milk

1 cup all-purpose flour

A pinch of salt

A pinch of grated nutmeg

A pinch of ground cloves

2 tablespoons olive oil

Directions

Place the yeast, sugar and 2 tablespoons of the lukewarm milk in a small mixing bowl; whisk

to combine and let it dissolve and ferment for about 10 minutes.

In a mixing bowl, combine the flour with the salt, nutmeg and cloves; add in the yeast mixture and stir to combine well.

Gradually pour in the milk and stir until everything is well incorporated. Let the batter sit for about 30 minutes at a warm place.

Heat a small amount of the oil in a nonstick skillet over a moderate flame. Drop the batter, 1/4 cup at a time, onto the preheated skillet. Fry until bubbles form or about 2 minutes. 5. Flip your blini and continue frying until brown, about 2 minutes more. Repeat with the\sremaining oil and batter,

6. Serve with toppings of choice. Bon appétit!

Old-Fashioned Cornbread\s(Ready in about 50 minutes | Servings 10)

Per serving : Calories: 388; Fat: 7g; Carbs: 39g; Protein: 7g

Ingredients\s2 tablespoons chia seeds

1 ½ cups plain flour

1 cup cornmeal

1 teaspoon baking powder

1 teaspoon baking soda

1 teaspoon kosher salt

⅓ cup sugar

1 ½ cups oat milk

⅓ cup olive oil

Directions

Start by preheating your oven to 420 degrees F. Now, spritz a baking pan with a nonstick

cooking spray.

To make the chia "egg", mix 2 tablespoons of the chia seeds with 4 tablespoons of the water. Stir and let it sit for about 15 minutes.

In a mixing bowl, thoroughly combine the flour, cornmeal, baking powder, baking soda, salt and sugar.

Gradually add in the chia “egg”, oat milk and olive oil, whisking constantly to avoid lumps. Scrape the batter into the prepared baking pan.

Bake your cornbread for about 25 minutes or until a tester inserted in the middle comes out dry and clean.

Let it stand for about 10 minutes before slicing and serving. Bon appétit!

Breakfast Banana Muffins with Pecans\s(Ready in about 30 minutes | Servings 9)

Serves: 1 Calories: 258; Fat: 7g; Carbs: 8g; Protein: 1g

Ingredients\s2 ripe bananas

4 tablespoons coconut oil, room temperature

2 tablespoons maple syrup

1/2 cup brown sugar

1 ½ cups all-purpose flour

1/2 teaspoon baking powder

1/2 teaspoon baking soda

1/2 teaspoon salt

1/4 teaspoon grated nutmeg

1/4 teaspoon ground cardamom

1/3 teaspoon ground cinnamon

1/2 cup pecans, chopped

Directions

1. Begin by preheating your oven to 350 degrees F. Coat 9-cup muffin tin with muffin liners. 2. In a mixing bowl, mash the bananas; stir in the coconut oil, maple syrup and sugar. Gradually

stir in the flour, followed by the baking powder, baking soda and spices.

Stir to combine well and fold in the pecans. Scrape the mixture into the prepared muffin tin.

Bake your muffins in the preheated oven for about 27 minutes, or until a tester comes out dry and clean. Bon appétit!

Grandma's Breakfast Gallete (Ready in about 40 minutes | Servings 5) Per serving : Calories: 208; Fat: 7g; Carbs: 7g; Protein: 8g

Ingredients 1 cup all-purpose flour

1/2 cup oat flour 1 teaspoon baking powder

1 teaspoon baking soda

1/2 teaspoon kosher salt

1 teaspoon brown sugar

1/4 teaspoon ground allspice

1 cup water

1/2 cup rice milk

2 tablespoons olive oil

Directions

Mix the flour, baking powder, baking soda, salt, sugar and ground allspice using an electric

mixer.

Gradually pour in the water, milk and oil and continue mixing until everything is well incorporated.

Heat a lightly greased griddle over medium-high heat.

Ladle 1/4 of the batter into the preheated griddle and cook until your galette is golden and crisp. Repeat with the remaining batter.

Serve your galette with a homemade jelly, if desired. Bon appétit!

Homemade Chocolate Crunch (Ready in about 35 minutes | Servings 9)

Per serving : Calories: 372; Fat: 9g; Carbs: 7g; Protein: 2g

Ingredients 1/2 cup rye flakes

1/2 cup buckwheat flakes

1 cup rolled oats

1/2 cup pecans, chopped

1/2 cup hazelnuts, chopped

1 cup coconut, shredded

1/2 cup date syrup

1 teaspoon vanilla paste

1/2 teaspoon pumpkin spice mix

1/4 cup coconut oil, softened

1/2 cup chocolate chunks

Directions

Start by preheating your oven to 330 degrees F. Line a baking sheet with parchment paper or

a Silpat mat.

In a mixing bowl, thoroughly combine all the Ingredients, except for the chocolate chunks. Then, spread the cereal mixture onto the prepared baking sheet.

Bake for about 33 minutes or until crunchy. Fold the chocolate chunks into the warm cereal mixture.

Allow it to cool fully before breaking up into clumps. Serve with a plant-based milk of choice. Bon appétit!

Chapter 2

SOUPS & SALADS

Classic Lentil Soup with Swiss Chard (Ready in about 25 minutes | Servings 5)

Per serving : Calories: 148; Fat: 2g; Carbs: 6g; Protein: 7g

Ingredients 2 tablespoons olive oil

1 white onion, chopped

1 teaspoon garlic, minced 2 large carrots, chopped 1 parsnip, chopped 2 stalks celery, chopped 2 bay leaves

1/2 teaspoon dried thyme

1/4 teaspoon ground cumin

5 cups roasted vegetable broth

1 ¼ cups brown lentils, soaked overnight and rinsed

2 cups Swiss chard, torn into pieces

Directions

In a heavy-bottomed pot, heat the olive oil over a moderate heat. Now, sauté the vegetables

along with the spices for about 3 minutes until they are just tender.

Add in the vegetable broth and lentils, bringing it to a boil. Immediately turn the heat to a simmer and add in the bay leaves. Let it cook for about 15 minutes or until lentils are tender. 3. Add in the Swiss chard, cover and let it simmer for 5 minutes more or until the chard wilts. 4. Serve in individual bowls and enjoy!

Spicy Winter Farro Soup (Ready in about 30 minutes | Servings 4) Per serving : Calories: 298; Fat: 9g; Carbs: 6g; Protein: 7g

Ingredients 2 tablespoons olive oil

1 medium-sized leek, chopped 1 medium-sized turnip, sliced 2 Italian peppers, seeded and chopped 1 jalapeno pepper, minced

2 potatoes, peeled and diced

4 cups vegetable broth

1 cup farro, rinsed

1/2 teaspoon granulated garlic

1/2 teaspoon turmeric powder

1 bay laurel

2 cups spinach, turn into pieces

Directions

In a heavy-bottomed pot, heat the olive oil over a moderate heat. Now, sauté the leek, turnip,

peppers and potatoes for about 5 minutes until they are crisp-tender.

Add in the vegetable broth, farro, granulated garlic, turmeric and bay laurel; bring it to a boil.

Immediately turn the heat to a simmer. Let it cook for about 25 minutes or until farro and potatoes have softened.

Add in the spinach and remove the pot from the heat; let the spinach sit in the residual heat until it wilts. Bon appétit!

Rainbow Chickpea Salad (Ready in about 30 minutes | Servings 4) Per serving : Calories: 378; Fat: 24g; Carbs: 2g; Protein: 1g

Ingredients

16 ounces canned chickpeas, drained

1 medium avocado, sliced 1 bell pepper, seeded and sliced 1 large tomato, sliced 2 cucumber, diced 1 red onion, sliced 1/2 teaspoon garlic, minced

1/4 cup fresh parsley, chopped 1/4 cup olive oil

2 tablespoons apple cider vinegar

1/2 lime, freshly squeezed Sea salt and ground black pepper, to taste

Directions

Toss all the Ingredients in a salad bowl.

Place the salad in your refrigerator for about 1 hour before serving. 3. Bon appétit!

Lentil Salad in the Mediterranean Style (Serves 5 | 20 minutes to prepare + chilling time) Serves: 1 348 calories, 15 grams of fat, 6 grams of carbohydrate, and 8 grams of protein

12 cup rinsed red lentils Ingredients

deli mustard (1 teaspoon)

freshly squeezed half a lemon

tamari sauce, 2 tblsp

1/4 cup extra-virgin olive oil 2 scallion stalks (chopped)

2 finely minced garlic cloves

1 cup torn-up butterhead lettuce

2 tbsp. chopped parsley

2 tbsp. chopped cilantro

fresh basil (1 teaspoon)

1 tsp oregano (fresh)

3 ounces 1 12 cup halved cherry tomatoes pitted and quartered Kalamata olives

Directions

1. Bring the water and red lentils to a boil in a large saucepan.
2. Reduce to a low heat and cook your lentils for another 15 minutes.

or until the vegetables are tender Drain the water and set aside to cool.

Toss the lentils with the remaining Ingredients in a salad bowl until thoroughly combined.

At room temperature or chilled, serve. Greetings!

Salad with Roasted Asparagus and Avocado (serves 4) Serves: 1 378 calories, 2 grams of fat, 6 grams of carbohydrates, and 8 grams of protein

1 pound trimmed, bite-sized asparagus

2 garlic cloves, minced 1 chopped white onion

1 thinly sliced Roma tomato

olive oil, 1/4 cup

balsamic vinegar (quarter cup)

1 tbsp mustard powder

2 tablespoons chopped fresh parsley 1 tablespoon chopped fresh cilantro 1 tablespoon chopped fresh basil Sea salt and black pepper to taste

1 pitted and diced medium avocado

a half-cup of pine nuts, roughly chopped

Directions

Preheat the oven to 420°F.

Arrange the asparagus on a parchment-lined roasting pan, tossing with 1 tablespoon of the olive oil.

Bake for 15 minutes, rotating the pan once or twice to ensure uniform cooking. Place it in your salad bowl after it has completely cooled.

Toss the asparagus, vegetables, olive oil, vinegar, mustard, and herbs together in a large mixing bowl. To taste, season with salt and pepper.

Toss everything together and serve with avocado and pine nuts on top. Greetings!

Creamed Green Bean Salad with Pine Nuts (serves 5)

Serves: 1 308 calories, 2 grams of fat, 6 grams of carbohydrates, and 8 grams of protein

2 medium tomatoes, diced 2 bell peppers, seeded and diced 1 12 pound green beans, trimmed

1/4 cup pine nuts, roughly chopped 1/2 cup vegan mayonnaise 4 tablespoons shallots, chopped

deli mustard (1 tablespoon)

2 tbsp basil leaves, chopped

2 tablespoons chopped fresh parsley 1/2 teaspoon crushed red pepper flakes Sea salt and freshly ground black pepper to taste

Directions

In a large saucepan of salted water, cook the green beans for 2 minutes or until they are just tender.

minutes.

Drain the beans and place them in a salad bowl once they have completely cooled. Combine the beans and the rest of the ingredients in a mixing bowl.

Season to taste with salt and pepper. Greetings!

Soup made with cannellini beans and kale (serves 5) 188 calories per serving; 7 grams of fat; 5 grams of carbohydrates; 1 gram of protein

1 tblsp olive oil (optional)

1 tsp. ginger (minced)

cumin seeds (1/2 teaspoon)

a chopped red onion

1 chopped and trimmed carrot

1 chopped and trimmed parsnip

2 finely minced garlic cloves

5 c. broth

2 cups kale, torn into pieces 12 ounces cannellini beans, drained

to taste with sea salt and black pepper

Directions

Heat the olive over medium-high heat in a heavy-bottomed pot. Now add the ginger and garlic to the pan and cook for a couple of minutes.

1 minute to 1 minute and a half to 1 minute and a half to one minute and a half

Add the onion, carrot, and parsnip and cook for another 3 minutes, or until the vegetables are just tender.

Continue to sauté for another minute, or until the garlic is fragrant.

Then, bring to a boil with the vegetable broth. Reduce the heat to a low heat and continue to cook for another 10 minutes.

Continue to cook until the kale wilts and everything is thoroughly heated, then fold in the Cannellini beans and kale. Season to taste with salt and pepper.

Serve immediately by ladling the soup into individual bowls. Greetings!

Creamy Mushroom Soup (serves 5)

308 calories per serving; 5 g fat; 8 g carbohydrates; 6 g protein

Ingredients

2 tbsp. safflower oil

20 ounces Cremini mushrooms, sliced 2 garlic cloves, minced 1 large shallot, chopped

flaxseed meal, 4 tblsp

5 c. broth

1 13 cup coconut milk (full fat)

1 bay leaf, to taste with sea salt and black pepper

Directions

In a stockpot over medium-high heat, melt the vegan butter. Cook the shallot for a few minutes once it's hot.

3 minutes, or until fragrant and tender.

Cook, stirring occasionally, until the mushrooms have softened, then add the garlic. Cook for another minute or two after adding the flaxseed meal.

Combine all of the remaining ingredients in a large mixing bowl. Allow it to simmer, covered, for another 5 to 6 minutes, or until the soup has slightly thickened.

Greetings!

Salad Panzanella (Authentic Italian Panzanella Salad | Serves 3)

Serves: 1 334 calories, 4 grams of fat, 3 grams of carbohydrates, and 3 grams of protein

3 cups artisan bread (1-inch cubes)

3/4 pound asparagus spears, trimmed and cut into bite-size pieces

4 tbsp olive oil (extra virgin)

a chopped red onion

lime juice, 2 tblsp.

deli mustard (1 teaspoon)

2 diced heirloom tomatoes, 2 medium heirloom tomatoes

Arugula, 2 cups

2 c. spinach, baby

2 seedsed and sliced Italian peppers

to taste with sea salt and black pepper

Directions

On a parchment-lined baking sheet, arrange the bread cubes. Preheat oven to 350°F (180°C).

Preheat the oven to 310°F and bake for 20 minutes, rotating the baking sheet twice during the baking process; set aside.

Preheat the oven to 420 degrees F and toss 1 tablespoon of olive oil with the asparagus. Roast for 15 minutes, or until crisp-tender.

In a salad bowl, combine the remaining ingredients; top with roasted asparagus and toasted bread.

Greetings!

Salad with Quinoa and Black Beans (serves 4) Serves: 1 433 calories, 3 grams of fat, 57 grams of carbohydrates, and 1 gram of protein

2 cup water Ingredients

16 ounces canned black beans, drained 1 cup rinsed quinoa

2 thinly sliced Roma tomatoes

1 cucumber, seeded and chopped, 1 red onion, thinly sliced

pressed or minced garlic cloves

2 seedsed and sliced Italian peppers

2 tbsp parsley 2 tbsp cilantro

olive oil, 1/4 cup

1 tbsp. lemon juice

1 TBS ACV

1 tsp dill weed (dried)

1 tsp. oregano (dried)

To taste, season with sea salt and black pepper.

Directions

Bring quinoa and water to a boil in a saucepan. Turn the knob right away.

Bring to a low boil and then reduce to a low heat.

Allow for a 13-minute simmer, or until the quinoa has absorbed all of the liquid; fluff with a fork and cool completely. Then, in a salad bowl, place the quinoa. 3. Toss together the remaining ingredients in the salad bowl. Greetings!

Rich Bulgur Salad with Herbs (serves 4) Serves: 1 408 calories, 3 grams of fat, 8 grams of carbohydrates, and 1 gram of protein

2 cup water Ingredients

bulgur 1 cup

12 oz. chickpeas, rinsed and drained

1 thinly sliced cucumber (Persian)

2 thinly sliced bell peppers (seeded)

1 thinly sliced jalapeno pepper, seeded

2 thinly sliced Roma tomatoes

1 thinly sliced onion (approximately 1 cup)

2 tbsp basil 2 tbsp parsley 2 tbsp mint 2 tbsp chives 4 tbsp olive oil

balsamic vinegar, 1 tblsp

lemon juice, 1 tablespoon

1 tsp. garlic powder (pressed)

To taste, season with sea salt and freshly ground black pepper

nutritional yeast, 2 tbsp

half a cup sliced Kalamata olives

Directions

Bring the bulgur and water to a boil in a small saucepan. Reduce the heat to a low-simmering temperature right away.

Allow for about 20 minutes of cooking time, or until the bulgur is tender and the liquid has almost completely evaporated. Spread on a large tray to cool after fluffing with a fork.

Combine the bulgur, chickpeas, cucumber, peppers, tomatoes, onion, basil, parsley, mint, and chives in a salad bowl.

Whisk the olive oil, balsamic vinegar, lemon juice, garlic, salt, and black pepper together in a small mixing bowl. Toss the salad to combine the dressing and the ingredients.

Serve at room temperature with a sprinkle of nutritional yeast on top and an olive garnish. Greetings!

Classic Roasted Pepper Salad (serves 3) Serves: 1 178 calories, 4 grams of fat, 8 grams of carbohydrates, and 4 grams of protein

6 bell peppers Ingredients

extra-virgin olive oil, 3 tblsp.

red wine vinegar, 3 teaspoons

3 finely minced garlic cloves

2 tablespoons chopped fresh parsley, to taste Sea salt and freshly cracked black pepper

red pepper flakes (1/2 teaspoon)

6 tablespoons coarsely chopped pine nuts

Directions

Broil the peppers for about 10 minutes, rotating the pan halfway through.

Cook until charred on all sides, about halfway through the cooking time.

To steam the peppers, cover them with plastic wrap. The skin, seeds, and cores should all be thrown away.

Toss the peppers with the remaining ingredients and slice them into strips. Put it in the fridge until you're ready to eat it. Greetings!

Winter Quinoa Soup (serves 4) Calories: 328 per serving; fat: 1 gram; carbohydrates: 1 gram; protein: 3 gram

2 tbsp olive oil (optional)

1 cup yellow squash, chopped 4 garlic cloves, pressed or minced 1 onion, chopped 2 carrots, peeled and chopped 1 parsnip, chopped 1 celery stalk, chopped

4 c. vegetable broth (roasted)

2 quarts crushed tomatoes

quinoa, 1 cup

to taste with sea salt and black pepper

Laurel of the bay

2 cup Swiss chard, torn into pieces after the tough ribs have been removed

2 tbsp. chopped parsley (Italian)

Directions

Heat the olive over medium-high heat in a heavy-bottomed pot. Now add the onion, carrot, and celery to the pan and cook until they are soft.

3 minutes or until the vegetables are just tender (parsnip, celery, and yellow squash).

Continue to sauté for another minute, or until the garlic is fragrant.

Bring to a boil after adding the vegetable broth, tomatoes, quinoa, salt, pepper, and bay laurel. Reduce to a low heat and cook for another 13 minutes.

Simmer until the Swiss chard wilts, then fold it in.

Serve garnished with fresh parsley in individual bowls. Greetings!

Green Lentil Salad (serves 5)

Serves: 1 349 calories, 1 gram of fat, 9 grams of carbohydrates, and 4 grams of protein

12 cup rinsed green lentils (approximately)

Arugula, 2 cups

2 cups shredded Romaine lettuce

1 c. spinach baby

a quarter cup of chopped basil

1 cup chopped shallots

2 finely minced garlic cloves

1/4 cup drained and chopped oil-packed sun-dried tomatoes

extra-virgin olive oil, 5 tblsp.

fresh lemon juice, 3 tblsp

to taste with sea salt and black pepper

Directions

1. Bring 4 12 cup water and the red lentils to a boil in a large saucepan. 2. Reduce the heat to a low heat and cook the lentils for an additional 15 to 17 minutes.

minutes, or until soft but not mushy. Drain the water and set aside to cool. 3. Toss the lentils with the remaining Ingredients in a salad bowl until well combined.

4. Serve cold or warm. Greetings!

Soup made with acorn squash, chickpeas, and couscous (serves 4)

Serves: 1 378 calories, 11 grams of fat, 1 gram of carbohydrate, and 9 grams of protein

2 tbsp olive oil (optional)

2 cups cream of onion soup 1 shallot, chopped 1 carrot, trimmed and chopped 1 stalk celery, chopped 1 teaspoon garlic, finely chopped 1 teaspoon rosemary, chopped 1 teaspoon dried thyme, chopped

2 c.

1 c. couscous (dried)

to taste with sea salt and black pepper

red pepper flakes (1/2 teaspoon)

drained 6 oz. chickpeas

2 tbsp lemon juice, freshly squeezed

Directions

Heat the olive over medium-high heat in a heavy-bottomed pot. Now add the shallot to the pan and cook it for a minute or two.

3 minutes or until the vegetables are just tender (carrot, acorn squash, and celery).

Continue to sauté for 1 minute, or until fragrant, adding the garlic, rosemary, and thyme.

Bring to a boil after adding the soup, water, couscous, salt, black pepper, and red pepper flakes. Reduce the heat to a low and continue to cook for another 12 minutes.

Continue to cook for another 5 minutes, or until the canned chickpeas are heated through.

Drizzle the lemon juice over the top and serve in individual bowls. Greetings!

Mom's Cauliflower Coleslaw (serves 4) Serves: 1 Calories: 280; Fat: 6g; Carbs: 8g; Protein: 3g

Ingredients

2 cups small cauliflower florets, frozen and thawed

2 cups red cabbage, shredded

1 cup carrots, trimmed and shredded

1 medium onion, chopped

1/2 cup vegan mayonnaise

4 tablespoons coconut yogurt, unsweetened

1 tablespoon yellow mustard

1 tablespoon fresh lemon juice

1/2 teaspoon cayenne pepper

to taste with sea salt and black pepper

Directions

In a salad bowl, toss the vegetables until well combined.

In a small mixing bowl, thoroughly combine the remaining Ingredients. Add the mayo

dressing to the vegetables and toss to combine well.

Place the coleslaw in your refrigerator until ready to serve. Greetings!

Decadent Broccoli Salad\s(Ready in about 10 minutes + chilling time | Servings 4)

Serves: 1 Calories: 417; Fat: 6g; Carbs: 3g; Protein: 7g

Ingredients\s2 pounds broccoli florets

1/4 cup sunflower seeds

1/4 cup pine nuts

1 shallot, chopped

2 finely minced garlic cloves

1 cup vegan mayonnaise

balsamic vinegar, 1 tblsp

1 tablespoon fresh lime juice

1 teaspoon mustard

To taste, season with sea salt and freshly ground black pepper

1/2 cup pomegranate seeds

Directions

In a saucepan, bring about 1/4 inch of water to a boil. Add in the broccoli florets. Cover and

steam the broccoli until crisp-tender or about 5 minutes.

Let the broccoli florets cool completely and place them in a salad bowl.

Add in the sunflower seeds, pine nuts, shallot, garlic, mayo, balsamic vinegar, lime juice, mustard, salt and black pepper. Toss to combine well.

Garnish with pomegranate seeds and serve well-chilled. Greetings!

Creamed Cavatappi and Cauliflower Salad\s(Ready in about 15 minutes + chilling time | Servings 4)

12 ounces cavatappi pasta

1 cup cauliflower florets

1/2 cup vegan mayonnaise

1 tablespoon fresh lemon juice

1 onion, chopped

2 finely minced garlic cloves

deli mustard (1 teaspoon)

2 medium tomatoes, sliced\s2 cups arugula, torn into pieces

Directions

Bring a large pot of salted water to a boil. Now, cook the pasta and cauliflower florets for about 6 minutes.

Remove the cauliflower with a slotted spoon from the water. Continue to cook your pasta for a further 6 minutes until al dente.

Allow the pasta and cauliflower to cool completely; then, transfer them to a salad bowl.

Then, add in the remaining Ingredients and toss until well combined.

Taste and adjust the seasonings; place the salad in your refrigerator until ready to use. Greetings!

French Green Bean Salad with Sesame and Mint

(Ready in about 10 minutes + chilling time | Servings 5)

Per serving : Calories: 338; Fat: 3g; Carbs: 2g; Protein: 13g

Ingredients

1 ½ pounds French green beans, trimmed

1 white onion, thinly sliced

2 garlic cloves, minced

Himalayan salt and ground black pepper, to taste

1/4 cup extra-virgin olive oil

2 tablespoons fresh lime juice

2 tablespoons tamari sauce

1 tablespoon mustard

2 tablespoons sesame seeds, lightly toasted

2 tablespoons fresh mint leaves, roughly chopped

Directions

Boil the green beans in a large saucepan of salted water until they are just tender or about 2

minutes.

Drain and let the beans cool completely; then, transfer them to a salad bowl. Add in the onion, garlic, salt, black pepper, olive oil, lime juice, tamari sauce and mustard. 3. Top your salad with the sesame seeds and mint leaves. 4. Bon appétit!

Chapter 3

Grandma's Creamy Soup

(Ready in about 40 minutes | Servings 4)

Per serving : Calories: 400; Fat: 3g; Carbs: 5g; Protein: 3g

Ingredients

2 tablespoons olive oil

1 shallot, chopped

4 large carrots, trimmed and sliced

4 large potatoes, peeled and sliced

2 garlic cloves, minced

1/2 teaspoon ground cumin

1/2 teaspoon mustard powder

1/2 teaspoon fennel seeds

Kosher salt and cayenne pepper, to taste

3 ½ cups vegetable broth

1 cup coconut milk

Directions

In a heavy-bottomed pot, heat the olive oil over medium-high heat. Once hot, sauté the

shallot, carrots and potatoes for about 5 minutes, stirring periodically.

Add in the garlic and continue sautéing for 1 minute or until fragrant.

Then, stir in the ground cumin, mustard powder, fennel seeds, salt, cayenne pepper and vegetable broth; bring to a rapid boil. Immediately reduce the heat to a simmer and let it cook for about 30 minutes.

Puree the soup using an immersion blender until creamy and uniform.

Return the pureed soup to the pot. Fold in the coconut milk and continue to simmer until heated through or about 5 minutes longer.

Ladle into four bowls and serve hot. Bon appétit!

Mexican-Style Chili Soup

(Ready in about 1 hour 15 minutes | Servings 4) Per serving : Calories: 498; Fat: 4g; Carbs: 9g; Protein: 3g

Ingredients

2 cups dry red beans, soaked overnight and drained

2 tablespoons olive oil

1 medium-sized leek, chopped

2 red bell peppers, chopped

1 chipotle chili pepper, chopped

2 cloves garlic, chopped

4 cups vegetable broth

1 bay laurel

1/2 teaspoon fennel seeds

1/2 teaspoon mustard seeds

1/2 teaspoon cumin seeds

Kosher salt and ground black pepper, to taste

1/2 cup salsa

3 heaping tablespoons fresh cilantro, chopped

2 ounces tortilla chips

Directions

Place the soaked beans in a soup pot; cover with a fresh change of the water and bring to a

boil over medium-high heat. Let it boil for about 10 minutes.

Next, turn the heat to a simmer and continue to cook for 45 minutes; reserve.

In the same pot, heat the olive over medium-high heat. Now, sauté the leek and peppers for approximately 3 minutes or until the vegetables have softened.

Add in the chipotle chili pepper and garlic and continue to sauté for 1 minute or until aromatic.

Then, add in the vegetable broth, bay laurel, fennel seeds, mustard seeds, cumin seeds, salt and black pepper and bring to a boil. Immediately reduce the heat to a simmer and let it cook for 10 minutes.

Fold in the reserved beans and continue to simmer for about 10 minutes longer until everything is thoroughly heated.

Ladle into individual bowls and serve with salsa, cilantro and tortilla chips. Bon appétit!

Wine and Lemon Braised Artichokes

(Ready in about 35 minutes | Servings 4)

Per serving : Calories: 228; Fat: 4g; Carbs: 3g; Protein: 2g

Ingredients

1 large lemon, freshly squeezed

1 ½ pounds artichokes, trimmed, tough outer leaves and chokes removed

2 tablespoons mint leaves, finely chopped

2 tablespoons cilantro leaves, finely chopped

2 tablespoons basil leaves, finely chopped

2 cloves garlic, minced

1/4 cup dry white wine

1/4 cup extra-virgin olive oil, plus more for drizzling

Sea salt and freshly ground black pepper, to taste

Directions

Fill a bowl with water and add in the lemon juice. Place the cleaned artichokes in the bowl, keeping them completely submerged.

In another small bowl, thoroughly combine the herbs and garlic. Rub your artichokes with the herb mixture.

Pour the wine and olive oil in a saucepan; add the artichokes to the saucepan. Turn the heat to a simmer and continue to cook, covered, for about 30 minutes until the artichokes are crisp- tender.

To serve, drizzle the artichokes with the cooking juices, season them with the salt and black pepper and enjoy!

Roasted Carrots with Herbs

(Ready in about 25 minutes | Servings 4)

Per serving : Calories: 217; Fat: 4g; Carbs: 4g; Protein: 3g

Ingredients

2 pounds carrots, trimmed and halved lengthwise

4 tablespoons olive oil

1 teaspoon granulated garlic

1 teaspoon paprika

Sea salt and freshly ground black pepper

2 tablespoons fresh cilantro, chopped

2 tablespoons fresh parsley, chopped

2 tablespoons fresh chives, chopped

Directions

Start by preheating your oven to 400 degrees F.

Toss the carrots with the olive oil, granulated garlic, paprika, salt and black pepper. Arrange

them in a single layer on a parchment-lined roasting sheet.

Roast the carrots in the preheated oven for about 20 minutes, until fork-tender.

Toss the carrots with the fresh herbs and serve immediately. Bon appétit!

Easy Braised Green Beans

(Ready in about 15 minutes | Servings 4) Per serving : Calories: 207; Fat: 5g; Carbs: 5g; Protein: 3g

Ingredients

4 tablespoons olive oil

1 carrot, cut into matchsticks

1 ½ pounds green beans, trimmed

4 garlic cloves, peeled

1 bay laurel

1 ½ cups vegetable broth

Sea salt and ground black pepper, to taste

1 lemon, cut into wedges

Directions

Heat the olive oil in a saucepan over medium flame. Once hot, fry the carrots and green beans for about 5 minutes, stirring periodically to promote even cooking.

Add in the garlic and bay laurel and continue sautéing an additional 1 minute or until fragrant.

Add in the broth, salt and black pepper and continue to simmer, covered, for about 9 minutes or until the green beans are tender.

Taste, adjust the seasonings and serve with lemon wedges. Bon appétit!

Braised Kale with Sesame Seeds

(Ready in about 10 minutes | Servings 4)

Per serving : Calories: 247; Fat: 9g; Carbs: 9g; Protein: 3g

Ingredients

1 cup vegetable broth

1 pound kale, cleaned, tough stems removed, torn into pieces

4 tablespoons olive oil

6 garlic cloves, chopped

1 teaspoon paprika

Kosher salt and ground black pepper, to taste

4 tablespoons sesame seeds, lightly toasted

Directions

In a saucepan, bring the vegetable broth to a boil; add in the kale leaves and turn the heat to a

simmer. Cook for about 5 minutes until kale has softened; reserve.

Heat the oil in the same saucepan over medium heat. Once hot, sauté the garlic for about 30 seconds or until aromatic.

Add in the reserved kale, paprika, salt and black pepper and let it cook for a few minutes more or until heated through.

Garnish with lightly toasted sesame seeds and serve immediately. Bon appétit!

Winter Roasted Vegetables

(Ready in about 45 minutes | Servings 4) Per serving : Calories: 255; Fat: 14g; Carbs: 31g; Protein: 3g

Ingredients

1/2 pound carrots, slice into 1-inch chunks

1/2 pound parsnips, slice into 1-inch chunks

1/2 pound celery, slice into 1-inch chunks

1/2 pound sweet potatoes, slice into 1-inch chunks

1 large onion, slice into wedges

1/4 cup olive oil

1 teaspoon red pepper flakes

1 teaspoon dried basil

1 teaspoon dried oregano

1 teaspoon dried thyme

Sea salt and freshly ground black pepper

Directions

Start by preheating your oven to 420 degrees F.

Toss the vegetables with the olive oil and spices. Arrange them on a parchment-lined

roasting pan.

Roast for about 25 minutes. Stir the vegetables and continue to cook for 20 minutes more.

Bon appétit!

Traditional Moroccan Tagine

(Ready in about 30 minutes | Servings 4)

Per serving : Calories: 258; Fat: 2g; Carbs: 31g; Protein: 1g

Ingredients

3 tablespoons olive oil

1 large shallot, chopped

1 teaspoon ginger, peeled and minced

4 garlic cloves, chopped

2 medium carrots, trimmed and chopped

2 medium parsnips, trimmed and chopped

2 medium sweet potatoes, peeled and cubed

Sea salt and ground black pepper, to taste

1 teaspoon hot sauce

1 teaspoon fenugreek

1/2 teaspoon saffron

1/2 teaspoon caraway

2 large tomatoes, pureed

4 cups vegetable broth

1 lemon, cut into wedges

Directions

In a Dutch Oven, heat the olive oil over medium heat. Once hot, sauté the shallots for 4 to 5

minutes, until tender.

Then, sauté the ginger and garlic for about 40 seconds or until aromatic.

Add in the remaining Ingredients, except for the lemon and bring to a boil. Immediately turn the heat to a simmer.

Let it simmer for about 25 minutes or until the vegetables have softened. Serve with fresh lemon wedges and enjoy!

Chinese Cabbage Stir-Fry

(Ready in about 10 minutes | Servings 3)

Per serving : Calories: 228; Fat: 7g; Carbs: 2g; Protein: 4g

Ingredients

3 tablespoons sesame oil

1 pound Chinese cabbage, sliced

1/2 teaspoon Chinese five-spice powder

Kosher salt, to taste

1/2 teaspoon Szechuan pepper

2 tablespoons soy sauce

3 tablespoons sesame seeds, lightly toasted

Directions

1. In a wok, heat the sesame oil until sizzling. Stir fry the cabbage for about 5 minutes. 2. Stir in the spices and soy sauce and continue to cook, stirring frequently, for about 5 minutes

more, until the cabbage is crisp-tender and aromatic.

3. Sprinkle sesame seeds over the top and serve immediately.

Sautéed Cauliflower with Sesame Seeds

(Ready in about 15 minutes | Servings 4)

Per serving : Calories: 217; Fat: 17g; Carbs: 2g; Protein: 1g

Ingredients

1 cup vegetable broth

1 ½ pounds cauliflower florets

4 tablespoons olive oil

2 scallion stalks, chopped

4 garlic cloves, minced

Sea salt and freshly ground black pepper, to taste

2 tablespoons sesame seeds, lightly toasted

Directions

In a large saucepan, bring the vegetable broth to a boil; then, add in the cauliflower and cook

for about 6 minutes or until fork-tender; reserve.

Then, heat the olive oil until sizzling; now, sauté the scallions and garlic for about 1 minute or until tender and aromatic.

Add in the reserved cauliflower, followed by salt and black pepper; continue to simmer for about 5 minutes or until heated through

Garnish with toasted sesame seeds and serve immediately. Bon appétit!

Green Bean Salad with Sesame and Mint (serves 5) (Ready in approximately 10 minutes Plus chilling time)

Serves: 1 338 calories; 3 grams of fat; 2 grams of carbohydrates; 13 grams of protein

1 12 pound French green beans, peeled and trimmed

1 finely sliced white onion

2 garlic cloves, to taste, Himalayan salt and black pepper, minced

a quarter cup of extra-virgin olive oil

lime juice, 2 tblsp.

tamari sauce, 2 tblsp

1 tablespoon mustard (optional)

2 teaspoons lightly toasted sesame seeds

2 teaspoons finely chopped fresh mint leaves

Directions

In a large pot of salted water, cook the green beans for 2 minutes or until they are just tender.

minutes.

Drain the beans and place them in a salad dish after they have totally cooled. Combine the onion, garlic, salt, black pepper, olive oil, lime juice, tamari sauce, and mustard in a large mixing bowl. 3. Sprinkle sesame seeds and mint leaves on top of your salad. 4. Welcome to the table!

Grandma's Creamy Soup (takes around 40 minutes to prepare | serves 4)

Calories: 400; fat: 3g; carbs: 5g; protein: 3g per serving

2 tbsp olive oil (optional)

4 big carrots, trimmed and sliced 1 shallot, chopped

4 big peeled and sliced potatoes

2 finely minced garlic cloves

1/2 teaspoon cumin powder

1/2 teaspoon powdered mustard

fennel seeds, 1/2 teaspoon

To taste, kosher salt and cayenne pepper

12 cup vegetable broth 3 12 cup vegetable broth

1 quart of coconut milk

Directions

Heat the olive oil in a heavy-bottomed saucepan over medium-high heat. Sauté the mushrooms once the pan is heated.

5 minutes, tossing occasionally, shallot, carrots, and potatoes

Continue to sauté for 1 minute, or until the garlic is fragrant.

Then add the ground cumin, mustard powder, fennel seeds, salt, cayenne pepper, and vegetable broth, and quickly bring to a boil. Reduce the heat to a low simmer and continue to cook for another 30 minutes.

Using an immersion blender, puree the soup until it is creamy and consistent.

Toss the pureed soup back into the pot. Stir in the coconut milk and cook for another 5 minutes, or until well cooked.

Serve immediately in four bowls. Greetings!

Mexican-Style Chili Soup (serves 4) (Ready in approximately 1 hour 15 minutes) Calories: 498; fat: 4g; carbs: 9g; protein: 3g per serving

2 cups dried red beans, soaked overnight and then drained

2 tablespoons extra virgin olive oil

2 red bell peppers, chopped 1 chipotle chile pepper, chopped 2 garlic cloves, chopped 1 medium-sized leek, chopped

4 c. vegetable stock

Laurel of the bay

fennel seeds, 1/2 teaspoon

a quarter teaspoon of mustard seeds

cumin seeds (1/2 teaspoon)

to taste kosher salt and crushed black pepper

a half cup of salsa

3 heaping teaspoons chopped fresh cilantro

tortilla chips, 2 oz.

Directions

In a soup pot, place the soaked beans, fill with new water, and bring to a boil.

Over medium-high heat, bring to a boil. Allow for a 10-minute boil time.

After that, reduce the heat to a low heat and cook for another 45 minutes; set aside.

Heat the olive oil in the same saucepan over medium-high heat. Sauté the leek and peppers for about 3 minutes, or until they've softened.

Continue to sauté for 1 minute, or until the chipotle chili pepper and garlic are fragrant.

Bring to a boil, then add the vegetable broth, bay laurel, fennel seeds, mustard seeds, cumin seeds, salt, and black pepper. Reduce the heat to a low level and continue to cook for another 10 minutes.

Stir in the saved beans and cook for an additional 10 minutes, or until everything is fully cooked.

Serve with salsa, cilantro, and tortilla chips in separate bowls. Greetings!

Braised Artichokes with Wine and Lemon (about 35 minutes | 4 servings)

Calories: 228 per serving; fat: 4 g; carbs: 3 g; protein: 2 g

Ingredients

1 big, freshly squeezed lemon

12 pound artichokes, trimmed, chokes and tough outer leaves removed

2 teaspoons finely chopped mint leaves

2 teaspoons finely chopped cilantro leaves

2 teaspoons finely chopped basil leaves

2 garlic cloves, minced

a quarter cup of dry white wine

1/4 cup extra-virgin olive oil, plus a little more to drizzle

To taste, season with sea salt and freshly ground black pepper

Directions

Fill a bowl halfway with water, then squeeze in the lemon juice. Put the cleaned artichokes in the basin and soak them fully.

Combine the herbs and garlic in a separate small bowl. Rub the herb mixture all over the artichokes.

In a saucepan, combine the wine and olive oil, then add the artichokes. Reduce to a low heat and cook, covered, for another 30 minutes, or until the artichokes are crisp-tender.

Drizzle the artichokes with the cooking juices and season with salt and black pepper before serving.

Roasted Carrots with Herbs (about 25 minutes to prepare | 4 servings)

Serves: 1 217 calories; 4 g fat; 4 g carbohydrates; 3 g protein

Ingredients

2 pound carrots, trimmed and lengthwise halved

4 tablespoons extra virgin olive oil

1 teaspoon garlic granules

paprika, 1 teaspoon

freshly ground black pepper and sea salt

2 tbsp. chopped cilantro

2 tbsp. chopped parsley

2 teaspoons chopped fresh chives

Directions

Preheat the oven to 400 degrees Fahrenheit.

Combine the carrots, olive oil, granulated garlic, paprika, salt, and black pepper in a mixing bowl. Arrange

Place them on a parchment-lined roasting sheet in a single layer.

Roast the carrots for approximately 20 minutes, or until fork-tender, in a preheated oven.

Toss the carrots with the fresh herbs just before serving. Greetings!

Chapter 4

Easy Braised Green Beans

(Serves 4) (Ready in 15 minutes) Calories: 207 per serving; fat: 5g; carbs: 5g; protein: 3g

Ingredients

4 tablespoons extra virgin olive oil

1 carrot, peeled and sliced into matchsticks

12 pound trimmed green beans

4 peeled garlic cloves

Laurel of the bay

12 CUP OF VEGAN BROTH

to taste with sea salt and black pepper

1 lemon, peeled and cut into wedges

Directions

In a saucepan, heat the olive oil over medium heat. Fry the carrots and green beans once the oil is heated.

Cook for 5 minutes, stirring occasionally to ensure consistent cooking.

Continue to sauté for another minute, or until the garlic and bay laurel are aromatic.

Add the stock, salt, and black pepper, and cook, covered, for another 9 minutes, or until the green beans are soft.

Serve with lemon wedges after tasting and adjusting spices. Greetings!

Sesame Seeds in Kale Braised

(Serves 4 | Ready in approximately 10 minutes)

Calories: 247 per serving; fat: 9 g; carbs: 9 g; protein: 3 g

1 pound kale, cleaned, rough stems removed, broken into pieces Ingredients 1 cup vegetable broth 1 pound kale, cleaned, difficult stems removed, torn into pieces

4 tablespoons extra virgin olive oil

6 sliced garlic cloves

paprika, 1 teaspoon

to taste kosher salt and crushed black pepper

4 teaspoons lightly toasted sesame seeds

Directions

Bring the vegetable broth to a boil in a saucepan; add the kale leaves and reduce the heat to low.

simmer. Cook for 5 minutes, or until the kale has softened; set aside.

In the same saucepan, heat the oil over medium heat. When the pan is heated, add the garlic and cook for approximately 30 seconds, or until fragrant.

Cook for a few minutes more, or until cooked through, adding the saved kale, paprika, salt, and black pepper.

Serve immediately with toasted sesame seeds as a garnish. Greetings!

Winter Roasted Vegetables (45 minutes to prepare | 4 servings) Calories: 255; fat: 14g; carbs: 31g; protein: 3g per serving

1/2 pound carrots, peeled and sliced into 1-inch slices

parsnips, 1/2 pound, sliced into 1-inch slices

1 cup celery, cut into 1-inch slices

1 pound sweet potatoes, peeled and cut into 1-inch slices

1 onion, peeled and sliced into wedges

olive oil, 1/4 cup

1 teaspoon crushed red pepper

1 teaspoon basil (dried)

1 teaspoon oregano, dry

1 teaspoon thyme, dry

freshly ground black pepper and sea salt

Directions

Preheat the oven to 420 degrees Fahrenheit.

Combine the veggies, olive oil, and spices in a large mixing bowl. Place them on a parchment-lined baking sheet.

pan for roasting

Preheat the oven to 350°F and roast for approximately 25 minutes. Stir in the veggies and simmer for another 20 minutes.

Greetings!

Traditional Moroccan Tagine (about 30 minutes to prepare | 4 servings)

Calories: 258; fat: 2g; carbs: 31g; protein: 1g per serving

3 tblsp. extra virgin olive oil

1 big chopped shallot

1 teaspoon peeled and minced ginger

2 medium carrots, trimmed and chopped 2 medium parsnips, trimmed and chopped 4 garlic cloves

2 medium peeled and sliced sweet potatoes

to taste with sea salt and black pepper

1 tsp. chili sauce

1 tsp. fenugreek seeds

a half teaspoon of saffron

1 teaspoon caraway seeds

1 lemon, sliced into wedges 2 big tomatoes, pureed 4 cups vegetable broth

Directions

Heat the olive oil in a Dutch oven over medium heat. Sauté the shallots for 4 to 5 minutes once the pan is heated.

minutes, or until vegetables are soft.

Then, for approximately 40 seconds or until fragrant, sauté the ginger and garlic.

Bring the other ingredients to a boil, except for the lemon. Reduce the heat to a low simmer right away.

Allow for a 25-minute simmer, or until the veggies have softened. Enjoy with fresh lemon slices on the side!

Chinese Cabbage Stir-Fry (Serves 3 | Ready in 10 minutes)

Calories: 228; fat: 7g; carbs: 2g; protein: 4g per serving

Ingredients

3 tblsp sesame seed oil

1 pound sliced Chinese cabbage

1/2 teaspoon powdered Chinese five-spice

to taste kosher salt

Szechuan pepper, 1/2 teaspoon

2 tblsp soy sauce (optional)

3 teaspoons lightly toasted sesame seeds

Directions

1. Heat the sesame oil in a wok until it sizzles. For approximately 5 minutes, stir fried the cabbage. 2. Add the spices and soy sauce and simmer for another 5 minutes, stirring often.

more, stirring occasionally, until the cabbage is crisp-tender and fragrant.

3. Drizzle sesame seeds on top and serve right away.

Cauliflower with Sesame Seeds in a Sauté

(Serves 4 | Ready in approximately 15 minutes)

Serves: 1 217 calories; 17 grams of fat; 2 grams of carbohydrates; 1 gram of protein

12 pound cauliflower florets 1 cup vegetable broth

4 tablespoons extra virgin olive oil

2 sliced scallion stalks

4 minced garlic cloves

To taste, season with sea salt and freshly ground black pepper

2 teaspoons lightly toasted sesame seeds

Directions

Bring the vegetable broth to a boil in a big saucepan, then add the cauliflower and simmer until tender.

6 minutes, or until fork-tender; set aside.

Then, heat the olive oil until it's hot, and then sauté the scallions and garlic for approximately 1 minute, or until they're soft and fragrant.

Stir in the saved cauliflower, salt, and black pepper, and cook for another 5 minutes, or until cooked through.

Serve immediately with toasted sesame seeds as a garnish. Greetings!

Sweet Mashed Carrots\s(Ready in about 25 minutes | Servings 4)

Per serving : Calories: 270; Fat: 8g; Carbs: 2g; Protein: 5g

Ingredients\s1 ½ pounds carrots, trimmed

3 tablespoons vegan butter

1 cup scallions, sliced

1 tablespoon maple syrup

1/2 teaspoon garlic powder

1/2 teaspoon ground allspice

Sea salt, to taste

1/2 cup soy sauce

2 tbsp. chopped cilantro

Directions

1. Steam the carrots for about 15 minutes until they are very tender; drain well. 2. In a sauté pan, melt the butter until sizzling. Now, turn the heat down to maintain an insistent

sizzle.

3. Now, cook the scallions until they've softened. Add in the maple syrup, garlic powder, ground allspice, salt and soy sauce for about 10 minutes or until they are caramelized. 4. Add the caramelized scallions to your food processor; add in the carrots and puree the\sIngredients until everything is well blended.

5. Serve garnished with the fresh cilantro. Enjoy!

Sautéed Turnip Greens\s(Ready in about 15 minutes | Servings 4) Per serving : Calories: 140; Fat: 8g; Carbs: 13g; Protein: 4g

Ingredients

olive oil, 2 tablespoons

1 onion, sliced

2 garlic cloves, sliced\s1 ½ pounds turnip greens cleaned and chopped

1/4 cup vegetable broth\s1/4 cup dry white wine

1 tsp. oregano (dried)

1 teaspoon dried parsley flakes

Kosher salt and ground black pepper, to taste\sDirections

In a sauté pan, heat the olive oil over a moderately high heat.

Now, sauté the onion for 3 to 4 minutes or until tender and translucent. Add in the garlic and continue to cook for 30 seconds more or until aromatic.

Stir in the turnip greens, broth, wine, oregano and parsley; continue sautéing an additional 6 minutes or until they have wilted completely.

Season with salt and black pepper to taste and serve warm. Greetings!

Yukon Gold Mashed Potatoes\s(Ready in about 25 minutes | Servings 5)

Per serving : Calories: 221; Fat: 9g; Carbs: 1g; Protein: 7g

Ingredients

2 pounds Yukon Gold potatoes, peeled and diced

1 clove garlic, pressed

Sea salt and red pepper flakes, to taste

3 tablespoons vegan butter

1/2 cup soy milk

2 tablespoons scallions, sliced

Directions

Cover the potatoes with an inch or two of cold water. Cook the potatoes in gently boiling

water for about 20 minutes.

Then, puree the potatoes, along with the garlic, salt, red pepper, butter and milk, to your desired consistency.

Serve garnished with fresh scallions. Greetings!

Aromatic Sautéed Swiss Chard\s(Ready in about 15 minutes | Servings 4) Per serving : Calories: 124; Fat: 7g; Carbs: 1g; Protein: 5g

Ingredients\s2 tablespoons vegan butter

1 onion, chopped

2 cloves garlic, sliced\sSea salt and ground black pepper, to season

1 ½ pounds Swiss chard, torn into pieces, tough stalks removed

1 cup vegetable broth

1 bay leaf

1 thyme sprig

2 rosemary sprigs

mustard seeds, 1/2 teaspoon

1 teaspoon celery seeds

Directions

In a saucepan, melt the vegan butter over medium-high heat.

Then, sauté the onion for about 3 minutes or until tender and translucent; sauté the garlic for

about 1 minute until aromatic.

Add in the remaining Ingredients and turn the heat to a simmer; let it simmer, covered, for about 10 minutes or until everything is cooked through. Greetings!

Classic Sautéed Bell Peppers\s(Ready in about 15 minutes | Servings 2)

Per serving : Calories: 154; Fat: 7g; Carbs: 9g; Protein: 5g

Ingredients

3 tablespoons olive oil

4 bell peppers, seeded and slice into strips

2 garlic cloves, chopped

Salt and freshly ground black pepper, to taste

1 teaspoon cayenne pepper

4 tablespoons dry white wine

2 tablespoons fresh cilantro, roughly chopped

Directions

In a saucepan, heat the oil over medium-high heat.

Once hot, sauté the peppers for about 4 minutes or until tender and fragrant. Then, sauté the

garlic for about 1 minute until aromatic.

Add in the salt, black pepper and cayenne pepper; continue to sauté, adding the wine, for about 6 minutes more until tender and cooked through.

Season to taste with salt and pepper. Top with fresh cilantro and serve. Greetings!

Mashed Root Vegetables

(Ready in about 25 minutes | Servings 5) Serves: 1 Calories: 207; Fat: 5g; Carbs: 1g; Protein: 3g

Ingredients\s1 pound russet potatoes, peeled and cut into chunks

1/2 pound parsnips, trimmed and diced

1/2 pound carrots, trimmed and diced

4 tablespoons vegan butter

1 tsp. oregano (dried)

1 tsp dill weed (dried)

1/2 teaspoon dried marjoram

1 tsp basil powder

Directions

Cover the vegetables with the water by 1 inch. Bring to a boil and cook for about 25 minutes

until they've softened; drain.

Mash the vegetables with the remaining Ingredients, adding cooking liquid, as needed.

Serve warm and enjoy!

Roasted Butternut Squash\s(Ready in about 25 minutes | Servings 4)

Serves: 1 Calories: 247; Fat: 5g; Carbs: 8g; Protein: 3g

Ingredients\s4 tablespoons olive oil

cumin powder (1/2 teaspoon)

1/2 teaspoon ground allspice

1 ½ pounds butternut squash, peeled, seeded and diced

1 tablespoon white wine, dry

2 tablespoons dark soy sauce

1 teaspoon mustard seeds

paprika, 1 tblsp.

to taste with sea salt and black pepper

Directions

Preheat the oven to 420°F. Toss the squash with the remaining

Ingredients .

Roast the butternut squash for about 25 minutes or until tender and caramelized.

Serve warm and enjoy!

Sautéed Cremini Mushrooms\s(Ready in about 10 minutes | Servings 4) Per serving : Calories: 197; Fat: 5g; Carbs: 8g; Protein: 3g

Ingredients

olive oil, 4 tablespoons

4 tablespoons shallots, chopped\s2 cloves garlic, minced\s1 ½ pounds Cremini mushrooms, sliced\s1/4 cup dry white wine

to taste with sea salt and black pepper

Directions

In a sauté pan, heat the olive oil over a moderately high heat.

Now, sauté the shallot for 3 to 4 minutes or until tender and translucent. Add in the garlic and

continue to cook for 30 seconds more or until aromatic.

Stir in the Cremini mushrooms, wine, salt and black pepper; continue sautéing an additional 6 minutes, until your mushrooms are lightly browned.

Greetings!

Roasted Asparagus with Sesame Seeds

(Ready in about 25 minutes | Servings 4)

Serves: 1 Calories: 215; Fat: 1g; Carbs: 8g; Protein: 6g

Ingredients\s1 ½ pounds asparagus, trimmed

4 tbsp olive oil (extra virgin)

to taste with sea salt and black pepper

1 tsp. oregano (dried)

1/2 teaspoon dried basil

1 teaspoon red pepper flakes, crushed

4 tablespoons sesame seeds

2 tablespoons fresh chives, roughly chopped

Directions

Start by preheating the oven to 400 degrees F. Then, line a baking sheet with parchment

paper.

Toss the asparagus with the olive oil, salt, black pepper, oregano, basil and red pepper flakes. Now, arrange your asparagus in a single layer on the prepared baking sheet. 3. Roast your asparagus for approximately 20 minutes.

4. Sprinkle sesame seeds over your asparagus and continue to bake an additional 5 minutes or until the asparagus spears are crisp-tender and the sesame seeds are lightly toasted. 5. Garnish with fresh chives and serve warm. Greetings!

Greek-Style Eggplant Skillet (Serves 4) (Ready in 15 minutes)
Calories: 195 per serving; fat: 1 g; carbs: 4 g; protein: 4 g

Ingredients

olive oil, 4 teaspoons

12 pound peeled and sliced eggplant

1 teaspoon minced garlic

1 tomato, smashed, to taste with sea salt and powdered black pepper

cayenne pepper (1 teaspoon)

1 tsp. oregano (dried)

a quarter teaspoon of bay leaf powder

2 oz. pitted and sliced Kalamata olives

Directions

In a sauté pan, heat the oil over medium-high heat.

Then, for approximately 9 minutes, or until just tender, sauté the eggplant.

Add the additional ingredients, cover, and simmer for another 2 to 3 minutes, or until everything is well cooked. Warm the dish before serving.

Chapter 5

Keto Cauliflower Rice

(Serves 5 | Ready in 10 minutes)

Calories: 135; fat: 5g; carbs: 2g; protein: 4g per serving

2 medium cauliflower heads (with stems and leaves removed)

4 tbsp olive oil (extra virgin)

4 squeezed garlic cloves

To taste, 1/2 teaspoon red pepper flakes, crushed sea salt, and powdered black pepper

1/4 cup coarsely chopped flat-leaf parsley

Directions

1. In a food processor, pulse the cauliflower with the Sblade until it's broken down into "rice." 2. In a saucepan over medium-high heat, heat the olive oil. When the pan is heated, add the garlic and sauté until it is fragrant.

1 minute or 1 minute and 1 minute and 1 minute and 1 minute and 1 minute and 1

Continue to sauté for another 7 to 8 minutes after adding the cauliflower rice, red pepper, salt, and black pepper.

Season with salt and pepper to taste, then top with fresh parsley. Greetings!

(Serves 4) Easy Garlicky Kale (Ready in approximately 10 minutes) Serves: 1 217 calories; 4 g fat; 1 g carbohydrate; 6 g protein

4 tblsp. extra virgin olive oil

12 pound fresh kale, rough stems and ribs removed, cut into bits 4 garlic cloves, chopped

1 quart vegetable stock

cumin seeds (1/2 teaspoon)

1 tsp. oregano (dried)

paprika, 1/2 teaspoon

1 teaspoon powdered onion

to taste with sea salt and black pepper

Directions

Heat the olive oil in a saucepan over a fairly high heat. Sauté the garlic for approximately a minute now.

1 minute, or until fragrant

In batches, add the kale and gradually add the vegetable broth, stirring to ensure equal cooking.

Reduce to a low heat, add the spices, and cook for 5 to 6 minutes, or until the kale leaves have wilted.

Warm it up and enjoy it!

Braised Artichokes with Lemon and Olive Oil (about 35 minutes | 4 servings)

Serves: 1 278 calories; 2 g fat; 27 g carbohydrates; 8 g protein

12 cup water 1 12 cup water 1 12 cup water 1 12 cup water 1 12 cup water 1 12 cup water

2 freshly squeezed lemons

2 pound artichokes, trimmed and chokes and tough outer leaves removed

1 bunch fresh parsley (Italian)

2 sprigs thyme

2 sprigs rosemary

bay leaves (two)

2 chopped garlic cloves

1/3 cup extra virgin olive oil

to taste with sea salt and black pepper

red pepper flakes (1/2 teaspoon)

Directions

Add the lemon juice to a basin of water. Clean the artichokes and place them in the basin.

ensuring that they are totally immersed

Combine the herbs and garlic in a separate small bowl well. Apply the herb mixture on your artichokes.

In a saucepan, combine the lemon water and olive oil; add the artichokes. Reduce to a low heat and cook, covered, for another 30 minutes, or until the artichokes are crisp-tender.

Drizzle the artichokes with the cooking juices and season with salt, black pepper, and red pepper flakes before serving. Greetings!

Roasted Carrots with Rosemary and Garlic (approximately 25 minutes | 4 servings)

Serves: 1 228 calories; 2 g fat; 8 g carbohydrates; 8 g protein

Ingredients

2 pound carrots, halved lengthwise after trimming

olive oil, 4 teaspoons

2 tbsp vinegar de champagne

4 garlic cloves, minced

2 rosemary sprigs, chopped

to taste with sea salt and black pepper

4 tablespoons chopped pine nuts

Directions

Preheat the oven to 400 degrees Fahrenheit.

Combine the carrots, olive oil, vinegar, garlic, rosemary, salt, and black pepper in a mixing bowl. Arrange

On a parchment-lined roasting sheet, arrange them in a single layer.

Roast the carrots for 20 minutes, or until fork-tender, in a preheated oven.

Serve the carrots right away with pine nuts as a garnish. Greetings!

Green Beans in a Mediterranean Style (Ready in 20 minutes | Serves 4)

Calories: 159; fat: 8g; carbs: 8g; protein: 8g per serving

2 tbsp olive oil (optional)

1 seeded and diced red bell pepper

12 pound green beans 4 minced garlic cloves

mustard seeds, 1/2 teaspoon

fennel seeds, 1/2 tsp.

1 teaspoon dill herb, dried

2 pureed tomatoes

1 cup celery cream soup

1 tsp Italian herb blend

cayenne pepper (1 teaspoon)

salt and black pepper, freshly ground

Directions

In a saucepan over medium heat, heat the olive oil. Fry the peppers and green onions once the oil is heated.

5 minutes, tossing occasionally to ensure that the beans are evenly cooked.

Continue to sauté for another minute, or until the garlic, mustard seeds, fennel seeds, and dill are aromatic.

Puree the tomatoes, add the cream of celery soup, Italian herb mix, cayenne pepper, salt, and black pepper to taste. Cover and continue to cook for another 9 minutes, or until the green beans are cooked.

Taste, season with salt and pepper, and serve warm. Greetings!

Roasted Garden Vegetables (about 45 minutes to prepare | 4 servings)

Serves: 1 311 calories; 1 gram fat; 2 gram carbohydrates; 9 gram protein

Ingredients

1 pound peeled and cut into 1-inch pieces butternut squash

4 peeled and cut into 1-inch pieces sweet potatoes

1/2 cup peeled carrots, sliced into 1-inch chunks

2 medium onions, peeled and sliced into wedges

olive oil, 4 teaspoons

1 tsp. garlic powder

paprika, 1 tblsp.

1 teaspoon rosemary (dried)

mustard seeds (1 teaspoon)

To taste, kosher salt and freshly ground black pepper

Directions

Preheat the oven to 420°F.

Combine the veggies, olive oil, and spices in a bowl and toss to combine. Place them on a parchment-lined baking sheet and arrange them.

Pan for roasting

Preheat the oven to 350 degrees Fahrenheit and roast for 25 minutes. Continue to cook for another 20 minutes, stirring occasionally.

Greetings!

Roasted Kohlrabi (about 30 minutes | 4 servings) Calories: 177; fat: 14g; carbs: 5g; protein: 5g per serving

1 pound peeled and thinly sliced kohlrabi bulbs

olive oil, 4 teaspoons

mustard seeds, 1/2 teaspoon

1 teaspoon seeds de celery

1 tsp marjoram (dried)

1 teaspoon minced garlic granules

to taste with sea salt and black pepper

nutritious yeast, 2 tbsp

Directions

Preheat the oven to 450 degrees Fahrenheit.

Toss the kohlrabi with the olive oil and seasonings until everything is well covered. Arrange the kohlrabi in a circular pattern.

on a parchment-lined roasting pan in a single layer

Bake the kohlrabi for 15 minutes in a preheated oven, then toss them and cook for another 15 minutes.

Serve immediately with a sprinkle of nutritional yeast on top of the steaming kohlrabi. Greetings!

Cauliflower with Tahini Sauce (Serves 4 | Ready in 10 minutes)

Calories: 217 per serving; fat: 13 g; carbs: 3 g; protein: 7 g

Ingredients

1 quart of water

2 pound florets of cauliflower

to taste with sea salt and black pepper

a third of a cup of soy sauce

tahini (5 tablespoons)

2 garlic cloves, chopped

lemon juice (two teaspoons)

Directions

1. Bring the water to a boil in a big saucepan, then add the cauliflower and simmer for around 15 minutes.

Drain, season with salt and pepper, and set aside for 6 minutes or until fork-tender. 2. Combine the soy sauce, tahini, garlic, and lemon juice in a mixing bowl. Serve with the sauce spooned over the cauliflower florets.

3. Welcome to the table!

Cauliflower Mash with Herbs (Takes around 25 minutes to prepare | Serves 4)

Calories: 167; fat: 13g; carbs: 3g; protein: 4g per serving

Ingredients

12 pound florets of cauliflower

vegan butter (four tablespoons)

4 garlic cloves, cut, to taste with sea salt and crushed black pepper

1/4 cup unsweetened plain oat milk

2 teaspoons finely chopped fresh parsley

Directions

Set aside to cool after steaming the cauliflower florets for around 20 minutes.

Melt the vegan butter in a skillet over medium-high heat, then sauté the garlic for approximately 1 minute, or until fragrant.

In a food processor, combine the cauliflower florets, sautéed garlic, salt, black pepper, and oat milk. Puree until all of the ingredients are fully combined.

Serve immediately with fresh parsley leaves as a garnish. Greetings!

Skillet with Garlic and Herb Mushrooms (Takes around 10 minutes to prepare | Serves 4)

Serves: 1 207 calories; 2 grams of fat; 7 grams of carbohydrates; 1 gram of protein

Ingredients: 4 tbsp. vegan butter

12 pound halved oyster mushrooms

3 garlic cloves, minced

1 tsp. oregano (dried)

1 teaspoon rosemary (dried)

1 teaspoon parsley flakes (dry)

1 tsp marjoram (dried)

1/2 cup white wine (dry)

To taste, season with kosher salt and black pepper.

Directions

Heat the olive oil in a sauté pan over medium-high heat.

Sauté the mushrooms for 3 minutes, or until the liquid has evaporated. Garlic should be included now.

Continue to fry for another 30 seconds or until fragrant.

Add the seasonings and sauté for another 6 minutes, or until the mushrooms are gently browned.

Greetings!

Pan-Fried Asparagus\s(Ready in about 10 minutes | Servings 4)

Per serving : Calories: 142; Fat: 8g; Carbs: 7g; Protein: 1g

Ingredients

vegan butter (four tablespoons)

1 ½ pounds asparagus spears, trimmed

1/2 teaspoon cumin seeds, ground\s1/4 teaspoon bay leaf, ground\sSea salt and ground black pepper, to taste

1 teaspoon fresh lime juice

Directions

Melt the vegan butter in a saucepan over medium-high heat.

Sauté the asparagus for about 3 to 4 minutes, stirring periodically to promote even cooking. 3.\sAdd in the cumin seeds, bay leaf, salt and black pepper and continue to cook the asparagus

for 2 minutes more until crisp-tender.

4. Drizzle lime juice over the asparagus and serve warm. Good appetite!

Gingery Carrot Mash\s(Ready in about 25 minutes | Servings 4)

Per serving : Calories: 187; Fat: 4g; Carbs: 1g; Protein: 4g

Ingredients

2 pounds carrots, cut into rounds

2 tablespoons extra virgin olive oil

1 teaspoon ground cumin

Salt ground black pepper, to taste

1/2 teaspoon cayenne pepper

1/2 teaspoon ginger, peeled and minced

1/2 cup whole milk

Directions

Preheat the oven to 400 degrees Fahrenheit.

Toss the carrots with the olive oil, cumin, salt, black pepper and cayenne pepper. Arrange

Place them on a parchment-lined roasting sheet in a single layer.

Roast the carrots in the preheated oven for about 20 minutes, until crisp-tender.

Add the roasted carrots, ginger and milk to your food processor; puree the Ingredients until everything is well blended.

Good appetite!

Mediterranean-Style Roasted Artichokes\s(Ready in about 50 minutes | Servings 4)

Serving size: Calories: 218; Fat: 13g; Carbs: 4g; Protein: 8g

Ingredients\s4 artichokes, trimmed, tough outer leaves and chokes removed, halved

2 freshly squeezed lemons

4 tbsp extra-virgin extra-virgin olive oil

4 cloves garlic, chopped

1 teaspoon fresh rosemary

1 teaspoon basil leaves

1 teaspoon fresh parsley

1 teaspoon oregano, fresh

Flaky sea salt and ground black pepper, to taste\s1 teaspoon red pepper flakes

paprika, 1 teaspoon

Directions

Start by preheating your oven to 395 degrees F. Rub the lemon juice all over the entire

surface of your artichokes.

In a small mixing bowl, thoroughly combine the garlic with herbs and spices

Place the artichoke halves in a parchment-lined baking dish, cut-side-up. Brush the artichokes evenly with the olive oil. Fill the cavities with the garlic/herb mixture.

Bake for about 20 minutes. Now, cover them with aluminum foil and bake for a further 30 minutes. Warm it up and enjoy it!

Thai-Style Braised Kale\s(Ready in about 10 minutes | Servings 4)

Per serving : Calories: 165; Fat: 3g; Carbs: 5g; Protein: 3g

Ingredients\s1 cup water

1 ½ pounds kale, tough stems and ribs removed, torn into pieces

2 tablespoons sesame oil

1 tsp. garlic powder, squeezed

1 teaspoon peeled and minced ginger

1 Thai chili, chopped

1/2 teaspoon turmeric powder

1/2 cup coconut milk

to taste kosher salt and crushed black pepper

Directions

In a large saucepan, bring the water to a rapid boil. Add in the kale and let it cook until

bright, about 3 minutes. Drain, rinse and squeeze dry.

Wipe the saucepan with paper towels and preheat the sesame oil over a moderate heat. Once hot, cook the garlic, ginger and chili for approximately 1 minute or so, until fragrant. 3. Add in the kale and turmeric powder and continue to cook for a further 1 minute or until\sheated through.

4. Gradually pour in the coconut milk, salt and black pepper; continue to simmer until the liquid has thickened. Taste, adjust the seasonings and serve hot. Good appetite!

Silky Kohlrabi Puree\s(Ready in about 30 minutes | Servings 4) Per serving : Calories: 175; Fat: 8g; Carbs: 5g; Protein: 1g

Ingredients\s1 ½ pounds kohlrabi, peeled and cut into pieces

vegan butter (four tablespoons)

To taste, season with sea salt and freshly ground black pepper.

a quarter teaspoon of cumin seeds

1/2 teaspoon coriander seeds

1/2 cup soy milk

1 teaspoon fresh dill

1 teaspoon fresh parsley

Directions

Cook the kohlrabi in boiling salted water until soft, about 30 minutes; drain.

Puree the kohlrabi with the vegan butter, salt, black pepper, cumin seeds and coriander seeds.

Puree the Ingredients with an immersion blender, gradually adding the milk. Top with fresh dill and parsley. Good appetite!

Creamed Sautéed Spinach\s(Ready in about 15 minutes | Servings 4)

Serving size: Calories: 146; Fat: 8g; Carbs: 1g; Protein: 3g

Ingredients\s2 tablespoons vegan butter

1 onion, chopped

1 teaspoon minced garlic

12 CUP OF VEGAN BROTH

2 pounds spinach, torn into pieces

to taste with sea salt and crushed black pepper

1/4 teaspoon dried dill

1/4 teaspoon mustard seeds

1/2 teaspoon celery seeds

cayenne pepper (1 teaspoon)

1/2 cup oat milk

Directions

In a saucepan, melt the vegan butter over medium-high heat.

Then, sauté the onion for about 3 minutes or until tender and translucent. Then, sauté the

garlic for about 1 minute until aromatic.

Add in the broth and spinach and bring to a boil.

Turn the heat to a simmer. Add in the spices and continue to cook for 5 minutes longer.

Add in the milk and continue to cook for 5 minutes more. Good appetite!

Aromatic Sautéed Kohlrabi\s(Ready in about 10 minutes | Servings 4) Per serving : Calories: 137; Fat: 3g; Carbs: 7g; Protein: 9g

Ingredients\s3 tablespoons sesame oil

1 ½ pounds kohlrabi, peeled and cubed

1 teaspoon minced garlic

1/2 teaspoon dried basil

1/2 teaspoon oregano, dry

to taste with sea salt and crushed black pepper

Directions

1. In a nonstick skillet, heat the sesame oil. Once hot, sauté the kohlrabi for about 6 minutes. 2. Add in the garlic, basil, oregano, salt and black pepper. Continue to cook for 1 to 2 minutes

more.\s3. Serve warm. Good appetite!

Classic Braised Cabbage\s(Ready in about 20 minutes | Servings 4)

Per serving : Calories: 197; Fat: 3g; Carbs: 8g; Protein: 4g

Ingredients

4 tablespoons sesame oil

1 shallot, chopped

2 minced garlic cloves

bay leaves (two)

1 quart vegetable stock

1 ½ pounds purple cabbage, cut into wedges

1 teaspoon crushed red pepper

Sea salt and black pepper, to taste

Directions

Heat the sesame oil in a saucepan over medium flame. Once hot, fry the shallot for 3 to 4

minutes, stirring periodically to promote even cooking.

Continue to sauté for another minute, or until the garlic and bay laurel are aromatic.

Add in the broth, cabbage red pepper flakes, salt and black pepper and continue to simmer, covered, for about 12 minutes or until the cabbage has softened.

Taste, adjust the seasonings and serve hot. Good appetite!

Sautéed Carrots with Sesame Seeds

(Serves 4 | Ready in approximately 10 minutes)

Serving size: Calories: 244; Fat: 8g; Carbs: 7g; Protein: 4g

Ingredients

1/3 cup vegetable broth\s2 pounds carrots, trimmed and cut into sticks

4 tablespoons sesame oil

1 teaspoon garlic, chopped\sHimalayan salt and freshly ground black pepper, to taste

cayenne pepper (1 teaspoon)

2 teaspoons chopped fresh parsley

2 tablespoons sesame seeds

Directions

In a large saucepan, bring the vegetable broth to a boil. Turn the heat to medium-low. Add in the carrots and continue to cook, covered, for about 8 minutes, until the carrots are crisptender.

Heat the sesame oil over medium-high heat; now, sauté the garlic for 30 seconds or until aromatic. Add in the salt, black pepper and cayenne pepper.

In a small skillet, toast the sesame seeds for 1 minute or until just fragrant and golden.

To serve, garnish the sautéed carrots with parsley and toasted sesame seeds. Good appetite!

Roasted Carrots with Tahini Sauce\s(Ready in about 25 minutes | Servings 4)

Serving size: Calories: 365; Fat: 8g; Carbs: 3g; Protein: 1g

Ingredients\s2 ½ pounds carrots washed, trimmed and halved lengthwise

4 tablespoons extra virgin olive oil

to taste with sea salt and crushed black pepper

Sauce:

4 tablespoons tahini

1 teaspoon garlic, pressed

2 tablespoons white vinegar

2 tblsp soy sauce (optional)

1 teaspoon mustard (deli)

1 teaspoon agave syrup

1/2 teaspoon cumin seed

1/2 teaspoon dill herb, dried

Directions

Preheat the oven to 400 degrees Fahrenheit.

Toss the carrots with the olive oil, salt and black pepper. Arrange them in a single layer on a

parchment-lined roasting sheet.

Roast the carrots in the preheated oven for about 20 minutes, until crisp-tender.

Meanwhile, whisk all the sauce Ingredients until well combined.

Serve the carrots with the sauce for dipping. Good appetite!

Roasted Cauliflower with Herbs\s(Ready in about 30 minutes | Servings 4)

Serving size: Calories: 175; Fat: 14g; Carbs: 7g; Protein: 7g

Ingredients\s1 ½ pounds cauliflower florets

1/4 cup extra virgin olive oil

4 cloves garlic, whole

1 tablespoon fresh basil

1 tablespoon fresh coriander

1 tablespoon fresh oregano

1 tablespoon fresh rosemary

1 tablespoon fresh parsley

to taste with sea salt and crushed black pepper

1 teaspoon crushed red pepper

Directions

Begin by preheating the oven to 425 degrees F. Toss the cauliflower with the olive oil and

arrange them on a parchment-lined roasting pan.

Then, roast the cauliflower florets for about 20 minutes; toss them with the garlic and spices and continue cooking an additional 10 minutes.

Warm the dish before serving. Good appetite!

Creamy Rosemary Broccoli Mash (Ready in about 15 minutes | Servings 4)

Serving size: Calories: 155; Fat: 8g; Carbs: 1g; Protein: 7g

Ingredients

1 ½ pounds broccoli florets

3 tablespoons vegan butter

4 cloves garlic, chopped

2 sprigs fresh rosemary, leaves picked and chopped

Sea salt and red pepper, to taste

1/4 cup soy milk, unsweetened

Directions

Steam the broccoli florets for about 10 minutes; set it aside to cool.

In a saucepan, melt the vegan butter over a moderately high heat; now, sauté the garlic and rosemary for about 1 minute or until they are fragrant.

Add the broccoli florets to your food processor followed by the sautéed garlic/rosemary mixture, salt, pepper and milk. Puree until all of the ingredients are fully combined. 4. Garnish with some extra fresh herbs, if desired and serve hot. Good appetite!

Chapter 6

Easy Swiss Chard Skillet

(Ready in about 15 minutes | Servings 4)

Per serving : Calories: 169; Fat: 1g; Carbs: 9g; Protein: 3g

Ingredients

3 tablespoons olive oil

1 shallot, thinly sliced

1 seeded and diced red bell pepper

4 garlic cloves, chopped

1 quart vegetable stock

2 pounds Swiss chard, tough stalks removed, torn into pieces

to taste with sea salt and crushed black pepper

Directions

In a saucepan, heat the olive oil over medium-high heat.

Then, sauté the shallot and pepper for about 3 minutes or until tender. Then, sauté the garlic

for about 1 minute until aromatic.

Add in the broth and Swiss chard and bring to a boil. Turn the heat to a simmer and continue to cook for 10 minutes longer.

Season with salt and black pepper to taste and serve warm. Good appetite!

Wine-Braised Kale (Ready in about 10 minutes | Servings 4)

Per serving : Calories: 205; Fat: 8g; Carbs: 3g; Protein: 6g

Ingredients 1/2 cup water

1 ½ pounds kale

3 tablespoons olive oil

4 tablespoons scallions, chopped

4 garlic cloves, minced

1/2 cup white wine (dry)

a quarter teaspoon of mustard seeds

to taste kosher salt and crushed black pepper

Directions

In a large saucepan, bring the water to a boil. Add in the kale and let it cook until bright, about 3 minutes. Drain and squeeze dry.

Wipe the saucepan with paper towels and preheat the olive oil over a moderate heat. Once hot, cook the scallions and garlic for approximately 2 minutes, until they are fragrant. 3. Add in the wine, flowed by the kale, mustard seeds, salt, black pepper; continue to cook, covered, for a further 5 minutes or until heated through. 4. Ladle into individual bowls and serve hot. Good appetite!

French Haricots Verts (Ready in about 10 minutes | Servings 4)

Per serving : Calories: 197; Fat: 5g; Carbs: 4g; Protein: 4g

Ingredients 1 ½ cups vegetable broth 1 Roma tomato, pureed 1 ½ pounds Haricots Verts, trimmed

4 tablespoons extra virgin olive oil

2 minced garlic cloves

1/2 teaspoon red pepper

a quarter teaspoon of cumin seeds

1/2 teaspoon oregano, dry

To taste, season with sea salt and freshly ground black pepper.

1 tablespoon fresh lemon juice

Directions

Bring the vegetable broth and pureed tomato to a boil. Add in the Haricots Verts and let it

cook for about 5 minutes until Haricots Verts are crisp-tender; reserve.

In a saucepan, heat the olive oil over medium-high heat; sauté the garlic for 1 minute or until aromatic.

Add in the spices and reserved green beans; let it cook for about 3 minutes until cooked through.

Serve with a few drizzles of the fresh lemon juice. Good appetite!

Buttery Turnip Mash (Ready in about 35 minutes | Servings 4)
Serving size: Calories: 187; Fat: 6g; Carbs: 14g; Protein: 6g

Ingredients

2 c. liquid

1 ½ pounds turnips, peeled and cut into small pieces

vegan butter (four tablespoons)

1 cup oat milk

2 fresh rosemary sprigs, chopped

1 tablespoon fresh parsley, chopped

1 teaspoon ginger-garlic paste

Kosher salt and freshly ground black pepper

1 teaspoon red pepper flakes, crushed

Directions

Bring the water to a boil; turn the heat to a simmer and cook your turnip for about 30

minutes; drain.

Using an immersion blender, puree the turnips with the vegan butter, milk, rosemary, parsley, ginger-garlic paste, salt, black pepper, red pepper flakes, adding the cooking liquid, if necessary.

Good appetite!

Sautéed Zucchini with Herbs (Ready in about 10 minutes | Servings 4)

Per serving : Calories: 99; Fat: 4g; Carbs: 6g; Protein: 3g

2 tblsp. extra virgin olive oil

1 onion, sliced

2 garlic cloves, minced 1 ½ pounds zucchini, sliced Sea salt and fresh ground black pepper, to taste

cayenne pepper (1 teaspoon)

1/2 teaspoon dried basil

1/2 teaspoon oregano, dry

1/2 teaspoon dried rosemary

Directions

In a saucepan, heat the olive oil over medium-high heat.

Once hot, sauté the onion for about 3 minutes or until tender. Then, sauté the garlic for about

1 minute until aromatic.

Add in the zucchini, along with the spices and continue to sauté for 6 minutes more until tender.

Season with salt and pepper to taste. Good appetite!

Mashed Sweet Potatoes (Ready in about 20 minutes | Servings 4) Per serving : Calories: 338; Fat: 9g; Carbs: 68g; Protein: 7g

Ingredients

1 ½ pounds sweet potatoes, peeled and diced

2 tablespoons vegan butter, melted

1/2 cup agave syrup

1 teaspoon pumpkin pie spice

A pinch of sea salt

1/2 cup coconut milk

Directions

Cover the sweet potatoes with an inch or two of cold water. Cook the sweet potatoes in gently boiling water for about 20 minutes; drain well.

Add the sweet potatoes to the bowl of your food processor; add in the vegan butter, agave syrup, pumpkin pie spice and salt.

Continue to puree, gradually adding the milk until everything is well incorporated. Good appetite!

Sherry Roasted King Trumpet (Ready in about 20 minutes | Servings 4)

Per serving : Calories: 138; Fat: 8g; Carbs: 8g; Protein: 7g

Ingredients 1 ½ pounds king trumpet mushrooms, cleaned and sliced in half lengthwise.

olive oil, 2 tablespoons

4 cloves garlic, minced or chopped

1/2 teaspoon dried rosemary

1/2 teaspoon dried thyme

1/2 teaspoon dried parsley flakes

1 teaspoon Dijon mustard

1/4 cup dry sherry

To taste, season with sea salt and freshly ground black pepper

Directions

Start by preheating your oven to 390 degrees F. Line a large baking pan with parchment

paper.

In a mixing bowl, toss the mushrooms with the remaining Ingredients until well coated on all sides.

Place the mushrooms in a single layer on the prepared baking pan.

Roast the mushrooms for approximately 20 minutes, tossing them halfway through the cooking.

Greetings!

Beetroot and Potato Puree (Ready in about 35 minutes | Servings 5) Per serving : Calories: 177; Fat: 6g; Carbs: 2g; Protein: 4g

Ingredients 1 ½ pounds potatoes, peeled and diced

1 pound beetroot, peeled and diced

2 tablespoons vegan butter

1/2 teaspoon deli mustard

1/2 cup soy milk

cumin powder (1/2 teaspoon)

paprika, 1 tblsp.

to taste with sea salt and black pepper

Directions

Cook the potatoes and beetroot in boiling salted water until they've softened, about 30 minutes; drain.

Puree the vegetables with the vegan butter, mustard, milk, cumin, paprika, salt and black pepper to your desired consistency.

Greetings!

Thai Stir-Fried Spinach (Ready in about 15 minutes | Servings 4)

Per serving : Calories: 147; Fat: 9g; Carbs: 7g; Protein: 1g

Ingredients

2 tablespoons sesame oil

1 onion, chopped 1 carrot, trimmed and chopped 1 Bird's eye chili pepper, minced 2 cloves garlic, minced 1 ½ pounds spinach leaves, torn into pieces

1/3 cup vegetable broth

2/3 cup coconut milk, unsweetened

Directions

In a saucepan, heat the sesame oil over medium-high heat.

Then, sauté the onion and carrot for about 3 minutes or until tender. Then, sauté the garlic and Bird's eye chili for about 1 minute until aromatic.

Add in the broth and spinach and bring to a boil.

Turn the heat to a simmer and continue to cook for 5 minutes longer.

Add in the coconut milk and simmer for a further 5 minutes or until everything is cooked through. Greetings!

Roasted Squash Mash (Ready in about 35 minutes | Servings 5) Per serving : Calories: 157; Fat: 7g; Carbs: 27g; Protein: 7g

2 tbsp olive oil (optional)

2 pounds butternut squash

1/2 teaspoon garlic powder

to taste with sea salt and black pepper

mustard seeds, 1/2 teaspoon

1/2 teaspoon celery seeds

A pinch of grated nutmeg

A pinch of kosher salt

2 tablespoons agave nectar

Directions

Preheat the oven to 420°F. Toss the squash with the remaining

Ingredients .

Roast the butternut squash for about 30 minutes or until tender and caramelized.

Then, in your food processor or blender, puree the roasted squash along with the remaining Ingredients until uniform and smooth.

Greetings!

Easy Zucchini Skillet (Ready in about 10 minutes | Servings 4)

Per serving : Calories: 137; Fat: 7g; Carbs: 2g; Protein: 7g

Ingredients\s2 tablespoons vegan butter

1 shallot, thinly sliced

1 teaspoon garlic, minced 1 ½ pounds zucchini, sliced Flaky sea salt and ground black pepper, to taste

paprika, 1 tblsp.

1/2 teaspoon cayenne pepper

1/2 teaspoon dried thyme

1/2 teaspoon celery seeds

1/2 teaspoon coriander pepper

nutritious yeast, 2 tbsp

Directions

In a saucepan, melt the vegan butter over medium-high heat.

Once hot, sauté the shallot for about 3 minutes or until tender. Then, sauté the garlic for

about 1 minute until aromatic.

Add in the zucchini, along with the spices and continue to sauté for 6 minutes more until tender.

Season to taste with salt and pepper. Top with nutritional yeast and serve. Greetings!

Sweet Potato Puree (Ready in about 25 minutes | Servings 5)

Per serving : Calories: 219; Fat: 9g; Carbs: 2g; Protein: 7g

Ingredients 2 pounds sweet potatoes, peeled and cubed

olive oil, 2 tablespoons

1 shallot, chopped

2 finely minced garlic cloves

1/4 cup coconut milk, unsweetened Sea salt and cayenne pepper, to taste

2 tablespoons fresh chives, roughly chopped

2 tbsp. chopped fresh parsley

Directions

Cover the sweet potatoes with an inch or two of cold water. Cook the sweet potatoes in gently boiling water for about 20 minutes; drain well.

Meanwhile, heat the olive oil in a cast-iron skillet and sauté the shallot for about 3 minutes until tender; add in the garlic and continue to sauté an additional 30 seconds or until tender.
3. Then, puree the potatoes, along with the shallot mixture, gradually adding the milk, to your desired consistency.

4. Season with salt and pepper to taste. Serve garnished with the fresh chives and parsley. Greetings!

Balkan-Style Satarash (Ready in about 25 minutes | Servings 4) Per serving : Calories: 199; Fat: 1g; Carbs: 6g; Protein: 9g

Ingredients

olive oil, 4 teaspoons

1 large onion, chopped 1 pound eggplant, peeled and diced 2 red bell peppers, seeded and diced 1 red chili pepper, seeded and diced

2 garlic cloves, minced 1 teaspoon paprika, slightly heaping 1 bay leaf Kosher salt and ground black pepper, to taste

1 large tomato, pureed ½ cup vegetable broth

Directions

Heat the oil in a large saucepan over medium-high flame.

Then, sauté the onion for about 3 minutes or until tender and translucent. Add in the eggplant and peppers and continue sautéing an additional 3 minutes.

Add in the garlic and continue to cook for 30 seconds more or until aromatic.

Add in the remaining Ingredients, cover and continue to cook for 15 minutes more or until thoroughly cooked. Warm food is best.

Classic Avocado Tartines (Ready in about 5 minutes | Servings 3)

Per serving : Calories: 384; Fat: 9g; Carbs: 6g; Protein: 3g

Ingredients

2 medium avocados, pitted, peeled and mashed

lime juice, 2 tblsp.

to taste with sea salt and black pepper

1/2 teaspoon red pepper flakes, crushed

6 slices whole-wheat bread, toasted

1 large tomato, sliced 3 tablespoons sesame seeds, toasted

Directions

1. Combine the mashed avocado with the lime juice, salt, black pepper and red pepper. 2. Spread the mixture onto the toast;

top with tomatoes and sesame seeds. 3. Thank you for your interest.

Classic Tomato Bruschetta (Ready in about 10 minutes | Servings 4)

Per serving : Calories: 155; Fat: 9g; Carbs: 7g; Protein: 5g

Ingredients

4 slices bread

2 tablespoons extra-virgin olive oil

1 clove garlic, halved

2 tomatoes, diced

1 tsp. oregano (dried)

1 tsp basil powder

to taste with sea salt and black pepper

Directions

Brush the bread slices with the olive oil and toast them in a skillet.

Now, rub the toasted bread on one side with halved garlic cloves.

Top with the tomatoes; sprinkle oregano, basil, salt and black pepper over everything. Greetings!

Tomato and Hummus Stuffed Avocados (Ready in about 5 minutes | Servings 4)

Serves: 1 Calories: 211; Fat: 5g; Carbs: 1g; Protein: 8g

Ingredients

2 avocados, pitted 2 tablespoons fresh lemon juice

2 medium tomatoes, diced

1 chili pepper, seeded and chopped

2 finely minced garlic cloves

4 tablespoons hummus

to taste with sea salt and black pepper

Directions

Drizzle the avocado halves with the lemon juice.

Fill your avocados with tomatoes, chili pepper, garlic and hummus. Season your avocados

with salt and black pepper.

Serve immediately. Greetings!

Summer Squash in a Mediterranean Style (35 minutes to prepare | 5 servings)

Calories: 145; fat: 1 gram; carbohydrates: 6 gram; protein: 5 gram per serving

2 lbs. peeled, seeded, and diced summer yellow squash

olive oil, 4 teaspoons

1 tsp. minced garlic

1 tsp. oregano (dried)

1 tsp basil powder

1 tsp. thyme (dried)

To taste, season with sea salt and freshly ground black pepper

2.2 oz. Pitted and sliced Kalamata olives

Directions

Preheat your oven to 360 degrees Fahrenheit (180 degrees Celsius). Combine the squash and the remaining ingredients in a large mixing bowl and toss well.

Except for the olives, all the ingredients are listed below.

Roast the squash until fork-tender, about 30 minutes.

Garnish with Kalamata olives and serve immediately. Greetings!

Braised Wax Beans with Herbs (serves 4)

Serves: 1 185 calories, 14 grams of fat, 1 gram of carbohydrate, and 6 grams of protein

12 pound wax beans, 1 cup water

olive oil, 4 teaspoons

minced garlic cloves (four)

peeled and minced 1/2 teaspoon ginger

1 tsp bay leaf powder

To taste, season with kosher salt and black pepper.

2 tbsp. chopped parsley (Italian)

2 tbsp basil leaves, chopped

Directions

Raise the temperature of the water to high. Cook for about 5 minutes, or until the wax beans are tender.

are crisp-tender and should be kept in the refrigerator.

Heat the olive oil in a saucepan over medium-high heat for 1 minute, or until the garlic, ginger, and ground bay leaf are fragrant.

Add the salt, black pepper, and the green beans that were set aside; cook for 3 minutes, or until fully cooked.

Garnish with basil and parsley. Greetings!

Tomatoes and Wine Braised Cabbage

(Servings 4 | Ready in 20 minutes)

Serves: 1 339 calories, 29 grams of fat, 4 grams of carbohydrates, and 1 gram of protein

Ingredients

olive oil, 4 teaspoons

1 carrot, thinly sliced and trimmed 1 medium red onion, chopped

1 slivered and diced bell pepper

1 tsp. minced garlic

bay leaf (one)

1 diced and seeded chipotle chili pepper

12 pounds cabbage, cut into wedges 1/4 cup vegetable broth

1 tomato, Roma, pureed

1 tablespoon white wine, dry

1 tsp cayenne 1 tsp basil (dried)

To season, season with sea salt and black pepper.

Directions

1. In a saucepan over medium heat, heat the olive oil. Fry the onion, carrots, and potatoes once the oil is hot.

4 minutes, stirring halfway through to ensure even cooking. 2. Add the garlic, bay leaf, and chili pepper and cook for 1 minute more, or until fragrant.

Add the cabbage, Roma tomato, wine, cayenne pepper, dried basil, salt, and black pepper to the broth.

Then, cover and continue to cook for another 13 minutes, or until the cabbage is soft and the liquid has thickened slightly. Individual bowls should be used to serve the food. Greetings!

Spicy Cauliflower Steaks (serves 4)

Serves: 1 366 calories, 1 gram of fat, 2 gram of carbohydrates, and 9 gram of protein

2 medium cauliflower heads, sliced into "steaks" lengthwise

olive oil (1/2 cup)

minced garlic cloves (four)

1 tsp. flakes de pimentón

cumin seeds (1/2 teaspoon)

1 tsp bay leaf powder

To taste, season with kosher salt and black pepper.

Directions

Preheat the oven to 400 degrees Fahrenheit (200 degrees Celsius). 1/4 of the butter should be brushed over the cauliflower "steaks."

Place them on a parchment-lined roasting pan with the olive oil and seasonings.

Mix the remaining 1/4 cup olive oil with the aromatics in a mixing bowl.

After 20 minutes of roasting, brush the cauliflower steaks with the oil/garlic mixture and cook for another 10 to 15 minutes.

Greetings!

Mediterranean-Style Sautéed Kale (serves 4)

222 calories per serving; 15 grams of fat; 1 gram of carbohydrates; 2 grams of protein

4 tblsp olive oil (optional)

2 garlic cloves, thinly sliced 1 small chopped red onion

12 pound kale, torn into pieces after tough stems have been removed

peeled and pureed 2 tomatoes

1 tsp. oregano (dried)

1 tsp basil powder

1 tsp rosemary powder

1 tsp thyme (dried)

To taste, season with sea salt and freshly ground black pepper

Directions

Warm the olive oil in a saucepan over a medium-high flame. Now add the onion and garlic to the pan and cook until they are translucent.

2 minutes, or until fragrant

Stir in the kale and tomatoes to ensure that everything is cooked evenly.

Reduce to a low heat, add the spices, and cook for 5–6 minutes, or until the kale leaves wilt.

Warm it up before serving.

GLUTEN-FREE RICE AND GLUTEN-FREE GLUTEN-

CPSIA information can be obtained
at www.ICGtesting.com
Printed in the USA
BVHW010025070422
633551BV00016BB/866